VEGETARIAN RECIPES FOR THE 5:2 FAST DIET

by Liz Armond

Revised Edition 2018

Published Great Britain:

© Copyright 2014 – Liz Armond
Revised - 2018

ISBN-13: 978-1500598594
ISBN-10: 1500598593

ALL RIGHTS RESERVED. No part of this publication may be reproduced or transmitted in any form whatsoever, electronic, or mechanical, including photocopying, recording, or by any informational storage or retrieval system without express written, dated and signed permission from the author.

TABLE OF CONTENTS

Introduction	1
The 5:2 Fast Diet	4
Some Essential Cookery Notes	10
Breakfasts	15
Some Simple Breakfast Ideas	16
A Couple of Quick & Easy Lunches	23
Less than 200 Calories	25
Easy Mixed Salad - 40 kcal	26
Vegetable & Citrus Soup - 80 kcal	28
Tomato & Red Pepper Soup - 95 kcal	30
Ratatouille - 105 kcal	32
Lentil & Spring Greens Soup - 110 kcal	34
Hungarian Vegetables - 115 kcal	36
Cauliflower Crumb Bake - 120 kcal	38
Mixed Salad & Avocado - 120 kcal	41
Potato Salad - 120 kcal	42
Low Calorie Hummus - 125 kcal	44
Split Pea & Carrot Soup - 125 kcal	46
Italian Aubergines - 135 kcal	48
Butternut Squash Soup - 150 kcal	50
Hearty Potato & Leek Soup - 150 kcal	52
Mini Cheese Soufflé - 150 kcal	54
Pea & Spinach Dahl - 159 kcal	56
Spicy Veggie Burgers - 170 kcal	58
Vegetable Curry - 181 kcal	60
Tomato & Courgette Bake - 185 kcal	62
Spicy Quorn Mince - 189 calories	64
Chilli Beans - 200 kcal	66
Less than 300 Calories	69

Leek & Bean Frittata - 215 kcal	70
Spinach & Mushroom Pie - 220 kcal	72
Mushroom Omelette - 255 kcal	76
Vegetable & Bean Stew - 260 kcal	78
Veggie Sausage & Lentil Pasta - 260 kcal	80
Sweet Potato Curry Wraps - 280 kcal	82
Mushroom Risotto - 284 kcal	84
Brown Rice & Vegetables - 285 kcal	86
Butternut Squash & Pea Stew - 285 kcal	88
Vegetable Risotto - 285 kcal	90
Five Bean Wrap - 294 kcal	92
Hearty Summer Salad - 294 kcal	94
Nutty Mushroom Pilaf - 298 kcal	96

Less than 400 Calories — 99

Vegetable Stew & Dumplings - 315 kcal	100
Pasta & Cherry Tomatoes - 325 kcal	102
Sweetcorn Soufflé - 325 kcal	104
Leek & Mushroom Bake - 330 kcal	106
Mixed Vegetable Bake - 330 kcal	108
Vegetarian Shepherd's Pie - 340 kcal	110
Vegetable & Quorn Stew - 345 kcal	112
Low Fat Pesto Tagliatelle - 350 kcal	114
Vegetarian Potato Curry - 350 kcal	116
Butternut Squash Risotto - 365 kcal	118
Golden Rice & Onions - 365 kcal	120
Mushroom Risotto - 365 kcal	124
Penne & Pepper Sauce - 375 kcal	126
Baked Veggie Bolognese - 385 kcal	128
Tofu & Noodles - 386 kcal	130
Mushrooms & Mustard Mash - 390 kcal	132
Vegetarian Chilli - 390 kcal	134

Courgette & Cheese Tart - 398 kcal	**136**
Calorie Counter	**139**
About the Author	**161**
Other Books by Liz Armond	**162**
One Final Thing	**163**

INTRODUCTION

Trying to lose weight can be difficult and finding something that works for you can be even harder. That's why the 5:2 Fasting, or Intermittent Fast, Diet will be the one for you. It is well known that dieting is so much easier when you have recipes that help you achieve your goals. Even though it is quickly becoming one of the most popular diets to lose and maintain weight loss, there are still only a few recipe books that are suited to the normal everyday meals that most people want.

This cookbook will not require tedious work, fancy ingredients, or anything else that you do not have to hand. The recipes here are low calorie and healthy, but they make use of many of the basics in your home.

This recipes use what is in your cupboard with the purchase of only a few inexpensive items that can be reused. It is designed for those who want to lose weight but don't want to be on a boring diet week after week after week. Because you only diet for 2 days instead of 7 you will hardly know you are on a diet at all.

I enjoy being creative with my food, and I urge you to do the same. For example, try adding a little more spice, extra vegetables or a different stock. As a bonus, I have included a calorie counter to help you swap ingredients in the recipes if you need to. This should ensure you stay within your calorie limit.

I opted to place the recipes by calorie portion, so you can calculate the number of calories you have remaining, and then jump to the section with the relevant count. This will inspire you to stay creative and still have the ability to switch your meals without going over your daily allowance. With the recipe count added at the beginning, you can plan entire menu days in advance to stay on track. There is also a recipe index for those who prefer to find meals based on what they are in the mood for that day.

I hope that you enjoy the recipes, and the experience of having food that is quick and easy to prepare. Finally, all the recipes included in this book are suitable for those not dieting in your family. You can add potatoes, rice, or pasta as desired and / or crusty bread.

Above all else, enjoy your food and the process of cooking it. You are only dieting for two days a week, so it is not necessary to stress yourself about it. However, you will find that over time, you will start noticing labels and calorie counts much more than you used to.

THE 5:2 FAST DIET

The 5:2 diet or Fast Diet or Intermittent Diet are just a few names given to a popular way of losing weight, so called because generally speaking you can eat as you would normally (whatever that is) on 5 days a week but on the other 2 days, known as fasting days you must restrict your food and drink intake.

The original diet was recommending that you to cut your calories from 2000 to 500 calories if you are a woman and from 2500 to 600 calories if you are a man. This was regardless of your current weight or how much you aim to lose.

But good news, Dr Michael Mosley has recently updated the diet and now says you can safely eat 800 calories a day and still lose weight. As part of this revised 5.2 plan, it is advised to have an earlier supper on the evening before your fasting day and then in the morning have a later breakfast. You will then be fasting for around 13 hours or more during the night.

It doesn't matter which days you choose to feed or fast, but it is recommended that the fasting days are not done together.

Personally, I like to fast Mondays and Thursdays every week and this works for us because I have time to organize meals and I also have the long weekend free of watching too much what I eat. Depending on the speed you wish to lose the weight you could even adjust the ratio of fasting to feeding days. For example, you could try a 6:1 or 4:3 and so on. When you have reached your ideal weight perhaps then is the time to only fast for one day a week to maintain your target weight, but for now let's assume you have a goal to reach, so we will a look at the normal 5:2 diet in more depth.

On fasting days, you can elect to consume all your calories in one go, or more usual to spread them throughout the day. Breakfast can either be a low-calorie count which means you can probably have a light lunch as well or you can skip it altogether. I found skipping breakfast worked better for me as it didn't kick start my juices first thing and I had no problem lasting until midday lunch.

I quite often forgot all about food and went to 1 or 2 o'clock before I realized I was getting hungry.

I don't think I could eat breakfast and then have nothing until my evening meal unless I was seriously fasting, meaning I was going without all food for that day. I cover this in more depth in my book 'The Fast Way to Lose Weight'

There is varying opinion on whether filling up at breakfast or snacking throughout the day is more effective for weight loss. You will find your own preferred method, I tried both and found that splitting my calories between lunch and dinner worked better for me but then I can manage to skip breakfast, but you may not be able to.

However, with the increased calorie allowance to 800 this is no longer a problem. You can still miss breakfast if this is your choice and have a bigger lunch or dinner, what ever suits you.

You can even stick to the 500 or 600 calories older diet and lose the weight a little faster.

Drink water, tea or coffee to fill your empty stomach but no sugar and watch your milk intake or you will be eating into your calories.

But please don't worry about going over the 500/600/800 calories by a little bit because when you do follow this eating plan you will be amazed at how you start to take notice of what you eat on your 'normal' days and will in fact eat less anyway.

You could try fizzy water or diet soda and some people have suggested chewing sugar free gum although I found that made me hungry.

On your 5 normal days you can eat whatever you like within reason. This is not carte blanch to load your system with unhealthy take out's or junk food. What you will find is that you are looking at packaging much more than you used to. You will be shocked at the number of calories in one chocolate biscuit, I know I was. If you think about the calories in that one biscuit and then think of the percentage that biscuit is of your 500/600/800 calorie allowance you quickly come to appreciate why that weight crept on in the first place. This doesn't mean you have to give them up, just be aware how much each one is and stop at one or two on your normal days.

Remember if the hunger pangs become too much, do something active like going for a walk. You can drink as much water as you like and this will fill you up too. Try a little honey or lemon juice in a glass of warm water, you will soon feel full until your meal is due.

If you are worried about the long-term effects on your body, contrary to what some people think, fasting can be a healthy way to lose weight. It can reduce levels of IGF-1 (insulin-like growth factor 1, which can lead to accelerated aging). It can also 'switch' on DNA repair genes as well as reducing blood pressure and lowering cholesterol and glucose levels.

A word of warning, it is not recommended for pregnant women or diabetics on medication. In fact, anyone who has health problems or has an existing medical condition is strongly advised to consult their GP first. This is not to say you can't follow this diet, it is just so it can be done under medical advice or supervision.

Finally, keep going by thinking to yourself that this is only for 2 days a week, you are not on a full blown 7 days a week diet for weeks on end or in some cases what seems forever.

Well that's all there is to it, simples!!

Finally, if you are interested in other methods of fasting, I do cover this in my book on losing weight through fasting called, **'The Fast Way to Lose Weight'**

Also if you find you are still wondering what to eat on your fasting day. I have put together a **Vegetarian Meal Plans & Recipe Book** in which I have taken recipes from this cookbook and given you 21 Days of Fasting Menus so you don't have to think what to cook. That' over 10 weeks of ready calculated diet day menus to make it even easier.

SOME ESSENTIAL COOKERY NOTES

The main recipes in this book are suitable for either lunches or dinners, depending on how you have decided to split your allowance on the fasting days. They are all tried and tested and I have attempted to give the menu for 1 serving where possible. Where this has proved difficult because of the ingredient quantities they will be for 2 or 4 servings.

If I have given ½ a can of beans or other split ingredients the remainder can be stored in the fridge or freezer for other recipes or used for a non-fasting day meal. This has not been a problem for me because my husband is also fasting, so I cook either 2 portions or 4 portions and freeze the excess. This is very handy when you want a quick lunch or dinner on your fasting days.

I do recommend that you cook as big a portion as possible, that way you always have a meal in the freezer or fridge. Let's face it; it will be easier on your fasting days if you are not surrounded by food ingredients waiting to be cooked...

The ingredients in this book are given in

the standard US measurements and the metric equivalent. You should choose one or the other, but do not mix. Where I have not given appropriate quantities, you can convert them using the table below.

Recipes use many different abbreviations. Here are some I have used in this book.

Recipe Abbreviations, Weights & Volumes
  Standard US
  tsp = teaspoon
  tbsp = tablespoon
  oz/s = ounce/ s
  lb/s = pound/s
  fl. oz. = fluid ounce

  Metric
  ml = millilitres
  ltr = liter/litre
  g = grams

Teaspoons and tablespoons are level measure.
  1 tsp = 5ml
  1 tbsp = 15ml

Volume conversions

⅛ tsp = 0.5 ml
¼ tsp = 1 ml
½ tsp = 2 ml
1 tsp = 5 ml
½ tbsp = 7 ml
1 tbsp = 3 tsp = 15 ml
2 tbsp = 1 fl oz = 30 ml
¼ cup = 4 tablespoons or 60 ml
⅓ cup = 90 ml
½ cup = 4 fl oz or 125 ml
⅔ cup = 160 ml
¾ cup = 6 fl oz or 180 ml
1 cup = 16 tbsp or 8 fl oz or 250 ml
1 pint = 2 cups or 500 ml
1 quart = 4 cups or 1 liter

Weight Conversions

½ oz = 15g
1 oz = 30g
2 ozs = 60g
3 ozs = 85g
¼ pound = 4 ozs = 115g
½ pound = 8 ozs = 225g
¾ pound = 12 ozs = 340g
1 pound = 16 ozs = 454g

Oven Temperature Conversions
200 F = 95 C
250 F = 120 C
275 F = 135 C
300 F = 150 C
325 F = 160 C
350 F = 180 C
375 F = 190 C
400 F = 205 C
425 F = 220 C
450 F = 230 C

Ovens vary so cooking times are only approximate. Always preheat your oven and for fan-assisted ovens reduce the temperature by 20°F or see the manufacturer's instructions for your oven.

Portion Sizes
Portion sizes are a general guide but are based on the calories given. Appetites are different but if you want to lose weight you must stick to the portion size.

Oil - Water Spray
Frying, even shallow frying is not recommended as it can add a lot of calories to any meal. You can make up a solution of 1-part oil to 8 parts water and store it in one of

those plastic bottles used as plant de-misters that you can get from any store or garden centre.

When you need to broil or dry fry, a few sprays of this solution is enough to lubricate the broiler wire or pan to stop the food sticking. Give the bottle a good shake before using and I recommend sunflower or rapeseed oil. You can even spray the food with this mixture to stop it drying out when you broil or oven frying.

Calorie Controlled Cooking Spray
These can be widely purchased now and are useful when you just want to coat a pan to stop food sticking, without swamping the food with oil or fat.

BREAKFASTS

Personally, I found it a lot easier to go without breakfast, but this is a matter of choice or your metabolism or your willpower. My partner must eat breakfast, or his sugar level drops and he feels a bit light headed. He usually has the porridge made with 50% milk/water with some stewed plums, apple or rhubarb and finds that this is more than enough to keep him going until lunchtime.

If you decide to have breakfast, because of the increased new allowance then you should consider having something more substantial in the morning.

SOME SIMPLE BREAKFAST IDEAS

PORRIDGE WITH GRAPES OR PLUMS OR HALF A BANANA

Serves 1- 136 calories a portion
Preparation - 2 minutes
Cooking - 3 minutes

- 30g/ 1¼ oz Porridge Oats
- 200ml/7 fl oz / 1 scant cup of skimmed milk and water mixed 50/50
- 50 gm/ 2oz grapes or 2 tbsp of stewed plums or rhubarb or half a banana
- A dribble of honey if needed but try to do without.

Method

In a large 3.5-pint jug or bowl, mix porridge oats with the water and microwave on high for 2 minutes, stir and microwave for a further minute, serve topped with **one** of the above fruits and the honey.

SCRAMBLED EGGS WITH VARIOUS FILLINGS

Serves 1 = 170 calories a portion
Preparation - 2 minutes
Cooking - 3 minutes

- 2 medium eggs
- 1 medium tomato
- 1 tsp of fresh herbs to taste
- pinch of chilli flakes (optional)

Method

Chop the tomato and microwave with the chilli flakes (optional) for about 45 seconds to heat. Cook your scrambled eggs how you like them but preferably not overcooked and just add the heated tomato at the end to serve.

You can also replace the tomato with either 100g mushrooms or 100g spring onions. Just slice and fry off in a small non-stick pan, with just a spray of oil and add to the scrambled egg.

This may not be satisfying for everyone, but if you really need to eat something rather than go without breakfast, then this makes a change from porridge.

FRUIT & YOGURT

Serves 1 - 140 calories a portion

- Half a small banana
- 170g/ 6oz pot fat free plain yogurt

Method
Just slice banana and add to yogurt

FRUIT PLATTER

Serves 1 - 100-120 calories a portion

Choose 250g / 9oz of your favourite fruit such as Pink or White Grapefruit, Pineapple, Raspberries, Peaches or Nectarines, Kiwi Fruit. <u>No Banana though</u>.

Method
Prepare and mix together your chosen fruits and then just weigh out 250 grams for breakfast on your fasting days. You can snack on the surplus on your other days if you like or save for your second day, will keep in fridge just fine

FRUIT FOOL

This breakfast recipe can be adapted to seasonal fruits that are easily available in the shops and cheaper when in season. Choose from any of the following but only use 50g of each.

Serves 1 - 45- 55 calories per serving
Preparation - 2 minutes
Choose 50g / 2oz of **ONE** of the following:
- blackberries - fresh peach sliced - raspberries - tinned rhubarb - strawberries
- 50g / 2oz 0% fat Greek yogurt

Method
Mash or chop the chosen fruit and fold into the Greek yogurt.

EGG WHITE OMELETTE

Serves 1 - 57 calories per serving
Preparation - 2 minutes
Cooking - 2 minutes

- 3 large eggs
- a few basil or other fresh herb leaves
- 3 sprays light sunflower oil

Method

Separate the eggs and save the yolks for a non-fasting day meal.

Whisk together the egg whites and a good helping of salt and pepper. Spray the oil into a non-stick pan and heat until the pan looks hot. Pour in the egg whites and cook until ready but not too dry. Serve at once with the herb leaves.

LOW CALORIE FRIED BREAKFAST

This is a bit of a cheats fry up but when you really fancy something a bit tastier on one of your fasting days then this will hit the spot. Most supermarkets have the vegetarian sausages.

Serves 1 - 178 calories per serving
Cooking- 10 minutes

- 1 vegetarian sausage
- 1 large egg
- 1 medium tomato halved

Method

Heat a non-stick frying pan until hot. Add the sausage and when it starts to release some fat or liquid, swish it around the pan to coat and then add the two tomato halves. Fry for about 2 minutes or until they are both starting to brown.

Turn the sausage and tomatoes over and move to one side of the pan. Crack the egg into the space and fry for another three minutes. If the egg is not fully cooked, pop a lid or splash guard on top to help it along and then just serve.

ANOTHER FRY UP

This includes baked beans which will bulk it up a little more.

Serves 1 - 194 calories per serving
Cooking - 5 minutes

- 1 vegetarian sausage
- 1 large egg
- 100g / 4oz reduced sugar and salt baked beans

Method

Heat a small non-stick frying pan on a medium heat and when hot, add the sausage to the pan. Fry until cooked before adding the egg and then cook until the egg is to your liking.

In the meantime, heat the baked beans in a small saucepan or better still microwave covered for 1 minute. Serve with the egg and sausage and enjoy.

A COUPLE OF QUICK & EASY LUNCHES

COTTAGE CHEESE ON CRACKERS OR RICE CAKES

Serves 1 – 109 calories a portion plus
Choose from the following
- Kallo Organic Rice Cakes – 30 calories per cake
- Ryvita Crackers for Cheese – 27 calories per cracker
- Jacobs Choice Grain Cracker – 33 calories per cracker
- 100g Reduced Fat Cottage Cheese

Method

Just choose the biscuit you would like to put your cottage cheese on and calculate how many you can eat within your daily allowance. Top with a sliver of cucumber or tomato, salt and pepper. I find 3 rice cakes, or 4 crackers are plenty for lunch.

POACHED EGGS WITH SPINACH

Serves 1 – 200 calories
Preparation - 5 minutes
Cooking - 10 minutes

- 1 bag fresh spinach
- 2 eggs
- A little olive oil

Method

Poach the eggs as you like them. I find those silicone poaching pods are great and always deliver a perfect egg. Rinse the spinach in a colander or sieve and pour a kettle of boiling water over it to wilt.

Drain off excess water by pressing into the colander or sieve with a potato masher or other flat tool. Place on warmed plate and top with poached eggs and season to taste.

You can use frozen spinach if more convenient, just defrost 200g naturally, squeeze excess water out and heat gently until warmed through

LESS THAN 200 CALORIES

EASY MIXED SALAD - 40 KCAL

You can have this salad for lunch or dinner. It is a staple of my fasting days and I will eat this for lunch with either a cold veggie sausage or a one egg omelette either hot or cold. I will also eat this salad on my non-fasting days with a bigger omelette because it is easy to make and very good to eat and keeps me off the bread and cakes.

Serves 1 - 40 calories
Preparation 5-10 minutes

- 1 tomato
- 2 sticks celery
- 6 thick slices of cucumber,
- 2 spring onions
- 1 tbsp of reduced fat salad cream (20cal)
- Squeeze of balsamic glaze

Method

If you like but you don't need to, peel the celery. Then chop or slice all salad ingredients. Stir salad cream into the prepared salad.

You can use mayonnaise if preferred but add another 50 calories. I have tried the low-calorie mayonnaise but because they have taken oil out to reduce the calories it is quite tasteless and dry. I much prefer salad cream, it has a lot more bite.

Drizzle over a little balsamic glaze for a bit more flavour.

VEGETABLE & CITRUS SOUP - 80 KCAL

This tasty soup is a real tummy filler for lunch or an afternoon snack. I suggest you make this in bulk and freeze in individual portions so that you have a ready prepared meal to hand.

Makes 6 portions – 80 calories per serving
***Suitable for freezing
Preparation - 20 minutes
Cooking - 25 minutes

- 500g / 1lb 2oz carrots
- 1 swede
- 2 onions
- 2 garlic cloves
- juice and zest of 1 orange
- 1½ litres / 2¾ pints vegetable stock
- 1 tbsp red wine vinegar
- 1 tbsp tomato paste
- bunch chives, chopped

Method

Peel and dice the carrots and swede. Chop the onions and crush the garlic.

Put the vegetables, garlic, tomato paste and vinegar into a large pan, pour over the hot vegetable stock and stir thoroughly.

Bring back to a simmer and cook on a low heat for 15- 20 minutes or until vegetables are cooked.

Stir in the orange juice and zest together with the chopped chives and serve in warm bowls for a delicious and filling lunch or afternoon snack.

****Try having a Warburton's thin or similar low-calorie bread or wrap, either toasted or fresh to dip in this soup, just add 100 calories.

TOMATO & RED PEPPER SOUP - 95 KCAL

This makes a great starter or a light lunch and is very easy to make.

Serves 4 - 95 calories per serving
***Suitable for freezing
Preparation - 10 minutes
Cooking - 30 minutes

- 2 red peppers
- 2 garlic cloves
- 1 medium onion
- 1 cal oil spray
- 400g / 14oz tin of chopped tomatoes
- 75g / 3oz potatoes

Method

De-seed and chop the peppers into chunks. Chop or dice the onion and the garlic. Peel and cut the potatoes into good sized chunks and keep in water until needed.

Heat a pan over a medium heat and spray with 5 pumps of oil, add the peppers, onion and garlic and allow them to cook for about 5 minutes until softened. Make sure you stir often so that they don't stick.

Add the tinned tomatoes and potatoes and using the tomato can as a measure use 2 cans full of water to cover.

Simmer the soup for about 20 minutes until the vegetables are done, then allow them to cool slightly and blend until smooth. Reheat and serve.

This makes 4 portions but can be frozen for another fasting day

RATATOUILLE - 105 KCAL

This dish can be served as a substantial evening meal as the ratatouille is only 105 calories per serving. You can have any of your vegetarian options such as sautéed Quorn pieces or tofu. You could even use it as a filling for a medium jacket potato which is 136 calories per 100g. Just check the weight of your potato. You could also add it to a two-egg crepe for your lunch or supper.

Serves 2 – 105 calories per portion for the ratatouille
Preparation - 10-15 minutes
Cooking - 20 minutes

- 1 medium onion
- 1 garlic clove
- 1 small green bell pepper
- 1 small yellow bell pepper
- 1 small aubergine/egg plant
- 1 medium courgette/zucchini
- 100g / 4oz button mushrooms
- 400g / 14oz can chopped tomatoes
- 2 tbsp tomato paste
- 1 tsp of dried mixed herbs

Method

Peel and chop the onion, trim, de-seed and dice both peppers and the courgette/zucchini. Halve the mushrooms, chop the garlic.

Put all vegetables into a pan and add the chopped tomatoes and tomato paste and stir well. Add the dried herbs, a tsp of sugar and plenty of seasoning.

Bring to the boil and simmer uncovered for 20 minutes.

LENTIL & SPRING GREENS SOUP - 110 KCAL

The lentils and greens make a colourful combination and the taste is not bad either. Alternate the choice of greens and spinach for variety.

Serves 2 - 110 calories
Preparation - 10 minutes
Cooking 30-35 minutes

- 100g / 3¼ oz green lentils
- 1 medium onion
- 2 cloves of garlic
- 1 cal spray oil
- 100g / 3¼ oz fresh spring greens or spinach
- 400ml / 13oz / 1¾ cups of vegetable stock or water

Method
Rinse the lentils under running water and cook them in fresh water for 10-15 minutes until just beginning to go soft. Drain and rinse again.

Peel and chop the onion and garlic. Put 5

sprays of oil in a large pan and cook the onion until soft but not burnt, then add the garlic and lentils.

Wash and chop the greens or spinach and add it to the pan gradually, allowing it to shrink down but keep stirring.

When all the greens or spinach are in, reduce it by about half, add enough liquid to cover and cook for about 15 minutes if spring greens, 10 minutes if using spinach.

Allow to cool slightly, blend, reheat and serve.

HUNGARIAN VEGETABLES – 115 KCAL

This is a very low-calorie dish that can be kept in the fridge and eaten for quick lunches on either fasting or non-fasting days.

Serves 4 – 115 calories per serving
Preparation - 10 minutes
Cooking - 20 minutes

- 1 onion
- 2 garlic cloves
- 1 red & 1 green pepper
- 3 portabella mushrooms
- 400g / 14 oz tin artichoke hearts in water
- 400g / 14 oz tin chopped tomatoes
- 1 tbsp rose harissa paste
- 1 tbsp paprika
- 1 tbsp tomato paste
- 300ml / 10 fl oz vegetable stock

Method

Roughly chop the onion and crush the garlic. De-seed the peppers and cut into 8 pieces. Quarter the portabella mushrooms, drain and quarter the artichoke hearts.

Spray a large non-stick pan and heat until hot. Add the onion and cook for 4 minutes until soft but not burnt. Add the peppers, mushrooms, garlic and artichokes and cook for a further 3 minutes until browned.

Stir in the harissa and tomato pastes and the paprika and cook for a further minute. Add the tin of tomatoes and the vegetable stock, bring to a simmer and cook for 10 minutes until thickened.

Serve at once.

CAULIFLOWER CRUMB BAKE - 120 KCAL

This is a very simple and economical dish to make and is also very low in calories.

Serves 4 - 120 calories per serving
***Suitable for freezing
Preparation - 25 minutes
Cooking - 10 minutes

- 2 courgettes/zucchini
- 3 garlic cloves
- 1 tsp dried basil leaves
- 1 medium cauliflower
- 60g / 2 oz fresh breadcrumbs
- 60g / 2oz half fat grated cheese

Method
Preheat oven to 220° C / 450°F / Gas 7
Quarter the courgettes/zucchini lengthways and slice into chunky pieces. Crush the garlic and break the cauliflower into large florets.

Fry the courgettes/zucchini in a large pan that has been oil sprayed and heated up for 3 minutes until slightly browned.

Add 1 tsp of dried herbs and 2 of the garlic cloves and cook for a further minute.

Add the tomatoes and 100 ml / 3½ fl oz boiling water and then the cauliflower florets. Season to taste and bring back to the boil, cover and simmer for 10 minutes until cauliflower is cooked.

Mix together the breadcrumbs, cheese, remaining herbs and garlic. Put the cauliflower mixture into an oven-proof dish and scatter the breadcrumb mixture on top. Spray with low calorie spray oil and bake for 10 minutes until top is golden.

*If freezing portions just put cauliflower mixture into suitable containers and the breadcrumb mixture into separate dishes. Defrost thoroughly and follow final step above.

NOTES

MIXED SALAD & AVOCADO - 120 KCAL

Serves 1 - 120 calories
Preparation - 5 minutes

- 60- 80gm bag mixed salad leaves or rocket
- 3 small tomatoes
- 1 small or half a medium ripe avocado
- Selection of fresh herbs such as basil, mint or chives (optional)

Method

Slice the tomatoes and shred the mixed salad. Mix with the herbs if using and divide between two bowls. Slice the avocado and lay on the salad.

POTATO SALAD - 120 KCAL

This potato salad can be made in bigger batches and served at lunch or dinner with your other chosen foods. At 120 calories a serving it makes a nice lunch with chopped tomato and 6 thick slices of cucumber (25kcal)

Makes 1 portion - 120 calories
Preparation - 10 minutes
Cooking - 20 minutes

- 125g / 4½ oz small new potatoes
- 1 tbsp low-fat mayonnaise
- 1 tbsp low-fat Greek yogurt
- ½ tsp Dijon mustard
- 3 spring onions
- ¼ of a cucumber

Method
Cut the potatoes into roughly 2cm chunks and bring to the boil in a pan of lightly salted water and cook for 10-15 minutes or until soft.

Mix together the low-fat mayonnaise and yogurt, add the mustard and mix it in well.

Drain the potatoes and put them in a large bowl. When they have cooled a little, stir in the mayonnaise mixture and leave to cool completely.

Chop the spring onions and cucumber and add them to the cold potato salad, mix well, season to taste and serve.

LOW CALORIE HUMMUS – 125 KCAL

Hummus is a great little snacking or lunch food. It is quite filling if you have 3 rice cakes at 30 calories each with a thin slice of cucumber or tomato on top.

Makes 4 portions - 125 calories per portion
Preparation 5-10 minutes
Cooking 5 minutes

- 1 x 400g/14oz tin chickpeas
- 2 cloves of garlic
- juice of 1 lemon
- 2 tbsp tahini

Method
Drain and rinse the chickpeas. Put them in a pan with fresh water and heat gently for about 5 minutes. Drain the chickpeas but keep some of the liquid and set aside.

Crush the garlic, place in a food processor with the chickpeas and lemon juice.

Add the tahini and a tablespoon of the cooking liquid and process until smooth, adding more liquid if necessary.

For dipping per person:
½ red pepper, de-seeded and sliced into batons

2 inches cucumber, cut into batons

½ carrot, peeled and cut into batons

SPLIT PEA & CARROT SOUP - 125 KCAL

This soup can be done in big batches as it's ideal for freezing and putting into individual portions.

Serves 4 – 125 calories per serving
***Suitable for freezing
Preparation - 35 minutes plus overnight soaking
Cooking – 1 - 1¼ hours

- 50g / 2oz yellow split peas
- 1 cal oil spray
- 1 small onion
- 1 garlic clove
- thumb size piece fresh ginger
- 1 red chilli
- 1½ tsp hot curry paste
- 225g / 8oz carrots
- 1 medium potato
- Chopped coriander to serve

Method

Soak the split peas overnight in twice their volume of cold water. Peel and chop the onion, potato, carrots and garlic. De-seed and chop the red chilli and grate the fresh ginger.

Drain the split peas and thoroughly rinse. Place in a large saucepan with 1.5 litres (2½ pints) of cold water and bring to the boil. Boil rapidly for 10 minutes then reduce the heat to a gentle simmer for a further 30 minutes.

Heat 5 sprays of oil in another saucepan and fry the onion, ginger, garlic and chilli for 10 minutes, stirring often until nicely browned but not burnt.

Add the curry paste, carrots and potatoes and mix well. Cook for a further 5 minutes giving an occasional stir.

Add this mixture to the cooked split peas, bring back to the boil and simmer for 35 minutes or until the vegetables and split peas are nicely cooked through and tender.

Allow to cool slightly then place in a food processor or use a hand blender and mash until fairly smooth. Re-heat soup, season to taste and serve straight away with the chopped coriander scattered on top.

ITALIAN AUBERGINES - 135 KCAL

This is a very low calorie but really filling lunch dish. You could also use is as a vegetable dish with some vegetarian alternative main dish or quiche. It can be left to go cold overnight in the fridge and eaten as a salad accompaniment.

Serves 4 - 150 calories per serving
***Suitable for freezing
Preparation - 20 minutes plus cooling
Cooking - 40 minutes

- 1 medium onion
- 500g / 1lb 2oz aubergine / eggplant
- 1 tsp dried mixed herbs
- 400g / 14 oz tin chopped tomatoes
- 1 tsp syrup
- 50g / 1¾ oz pitted green or black olives
- 1 tsp red wine vinegar

Method

Slice the onion finely, dice the aubergine/eggplant, rinse and chop the olives.

Spray a frying pan with the cooking spray and fry the onion for roughly 3-4 minutes until soft. Add the chopped aubergine/eggplant and dried mixed herbs and cook for another 5-6 minutes, turning often.

Add the rest of the ingredients, bring to the boil and cover and simmer for 35 minutes. Add salt and pepper to taste.

BUTTERNUT SQUASH SOUP – 150 KCAL

This is a thick and warming soup that can be stored or frozen for another fasting day.

Serves 4 - 150 calories a portion
***Suitable for freezing
Preparation - 10-15 minutes
Cooking - 25-30 minutes

- 1 cal oil spray
- 1 small onion, chopped
- 1 clove of garlic, chopped
- 1 small butternut squash – about 250g / 9oz
- 1 litre / 1¾ pints / 4 cups of vegetable stock
- 1 pinch cayenne pepper

Method
Heat 5 sprays of oil in a large pan. Add the onion and garlic and cook very gently for about 5 minutes until translucent and sticky but not burnt.

Prepare the squash by cutting into quarters; take out the seeds and then peel.

Cut the remaining flesh into small chunks and when onion is ready, add the squash to the pan.

Stir, add the stock and cayenne pepper and bring to a low simmer. Lower the heat and cook for about 20 minutes.

When ready, leave to cool slightly and either use a blender or mash it by hand. Add a little more hot stock or water if the soup is too thick.

HEARTY POTATO & LEEK SOUP - 150 KCAL

This soup is so delicious, you really should make bigger batches of it and freeze for convenience.

Serves 1 - 150 calories a portion
***Suitable for freezing
Preparation - 15 minutes
Cooking - 45 minutes

- 100g / 3½ oz potatoes
- 250g/8oz small leeks, untrimmed
- 1 cal oil spray
- A few sprigs of Tarragon, stalks removed
- 80ml / 3 fl oz / ⅓ cup of skimmed milk

Method

Trim the leeks, cut into thin slices and place in cold water to get rid of any soil.

Peel and cut the potatoes into 2cm cubes. Heat 5 sprays of oil in a large pan over a medium heat.

Thoroughly drain the leeks and add to the pan. Cook gently for about 5 minutes. Add the potatoes and tarragon leaves and enough water to cover. Cook the vegetables for 15-20 minutes with the lid on, then add the milk and cook for another 20 minutes, adding more water if necessary.

Take out about ¼ of the soup including some potatoes and mash or whiz smooth. Return to the pan, season to taste and serve hot.

MINI CHEESE SOUFFLé - 150 KCAL

You can have these delicious cheese pots as a starter or better still for lunch with a green salad or steamed spinach.

Serves 2 - 143 calories per serving
Preparation - 15 minutes
Cooking - 15 minutes

- 40g / 1½ oz fresh breadcrumbs
- 1 egg
- 1 tsp wholegrain mustard
- 100ml / 3½ oz skimmed milk
- 40g / 1½ oz cheddar cheese

Method
Preheat oven to 190°C / 375° F / Gas Mark 5

Beat the eggs and grate the cheese.

Mix all the ingredients together, season with salt and freshly ground pepper and divide between 2 ramekin dishes. Leave to stand for 5 minutes.

When oven is ready, bake for 15 minutes until the soufflé has risen slightly. Serve at once with the salad or steamed broccoli.

PEA & SPINACH DAHL - 159 KCAL

This dish will warm and fill you up on your fasting day, what more could you want?

Serves 4- 159 calories per serving
***Suitable for freezing
Preparation - 10 minutes
Cooking - 50 minutes

- 1 large onion
- 4 cloves garlic
- 1 thumb size piece fresh ginger
- 1 large red chilli
- 1 cal oil spray
- 225g / 8oz red lentils
- ¼ turmeric powder and cayenne pepper
- 1 tsp paprika
- ½ tsp ground cumin
- 1200ml / 2 pints water
- 1 tomato
- juice of 1 lime
- 2 tbsp frozen peas
- 3 cubes frozen spinach

Method

Peel and roughly chop the onion, garlic and ginger. Do the same to the chilli but if you don't want it too hot you can remove all or some of the seeds and membrane.

Heat 5 sprays of the oil in a large heavy based pan and sauté all chopped ingredients for about 5 minutes or until the onion has softened. Add all the ground spices and fry for another couple of minutes stirring well.

Rinse the lentils in a sieve under cold running water for at least a minute and add them to the pan. Stir really well and then add the water and bring back to a boil. Boil at a steady rate for 10 minutes and then turn the heat down to a low simmer.

Continue to simmer at the lowest heat for about 30 to 40 minutes, making sure you stir the Dahl often to stop it sticking on the bottom of the pan. The mixture will thicken as it cooks and when it looks like thick rice pudding, add the spinach, peas, lime juice and the chopped tomato and cook for another 5 minutes and then serve in warmed bowls.

SPICY VEGGIE BURGERS - 170 KCAL

These vegetable burgers are super easy to make and are delicious served with a green salad of your choice and a chopped tomato with low calorie dressing.

Serves 2 - 170 calories per serving
Preparation - 10 minutes
Cooking - 40 minutes

- 200g / 7oz butternut squash
- 200g / 7 oz potatoes
- 1 egg
- ½ tsp ground cumin
- ½ tsp chilli powder
- 1 tbsp chopped flat leaf parsley
- 2 spring onions

Method

Peel, de-seed and dice the butternut squash, peel and dice the potatoes and finely slice the spring onions.

Bring a large pan of water to the boil and add the squash and potatoes. Bring back to a boil, cover and simmer for 10 minutes or until both are tender. At the same time boil the egg in a small saucepan of boiling water for the same time, remove from the heat and run under cold water.

Drain the squash and potatoes, rinse in cold water to stop them overcooking and drain again when cold. Return to the pan and mash or put through a potato ricer until smooth.

Peel the egg and roughly chop, then add to the squash mixture together with the spices, onions and parsley. Season well to taste and shape into 4 small burgers.

Heat a non-stick pan, spray with a low-calorie cooking spray and cook gently for 4-5 minutes until golden brown making sure you turn a couple of times to avoid burning.

Serve with a green salad, 1 chopped tomato and a sprinkling of chilli flakes if liked.

VEGETABLE CURRY – 181 KCAL

You could use a ready mixed madras curry powder instead of the spices. This could also be made in bigger portions and frozen. You could also use fresh vegetables, adjust the cooking time to make sure they are cooked before serving the curry.

Serves 1 - 181 calories per serving
***Suitable for freezing
Preparation 5 minutes
Cooking 40 minutes

- 1 cal oil spray
- ½ tsp cumin seeds & ½ tsp mustard seeds
- ½ onion
- 1 clove garlic
- ¼ tsp ground coriander & ¼ tsp ground cumin
- ¼ tsp turmeric
- ½ tsp mild chilli powder
- ½ tsp salt
- ½ tin chopped tomatoes
- 2 handfuls of pre-chopped frozen vegetables (choose from carrot, peas,

green beans, cauliflower, or anything else you like!)

Method

Finely chop the onion and garlic. Heat 5 sprays of the oil and cook the cumin and mustard seeds until the spices start to pop but do not burn them. Add the chopped onion and garlic, stir and lower the heat to a simmer. Cook the onions for about 10 minutes until they are translucent and starting to go brown.

Add the remaining spices and the salt, stir thoroughly and then add the chopped tomatoes. Add your choice of vegetables and then simmer gently for ½ an hour adding a little water if mixture starts to dry out.

TOMATO & COURGETTE BAKE - 185 KCAL

A tasty and very low-calorie dish to use as a main course or as an accompaniment for a veggie main dish.

Serves 4 - 185 calories a portion
Preparation - 10-15 minutes
Cooking - 30 - 35minutes

- 500g courgettes/zucchini
- 1 clove of garlic
- 400g tomatoes
- 2 tbsp green basil pesto
- 4 tbsp fresh breadcrumbs
- 25g mature cheddar

Method
Pre-heat the oven to 220° or Gas 7
Top and tail then thinly slice the courgettes/zucchini. Slice the tomatoes and grate the cheese.
Mix the courgette/zucchini slices and pesto sauce until lightly coated.

Arrange the courgette/zucchini and tomato slices in a single layer in a 2 litre oven proof dish and season well.

In a separate bowl mix together the breadcrumbs, finely chopped garlic and cayenne pepper and cover the vegetables with this mixture. Drizzle with a little olive oil.

Bake for 30 minutes until golden on top and the vegetables are cooked.

SPICY QUORN MINCE – 189 CALORIES

Serves 4 – 195 calories per serving
***Suitable for freezing
Preparation - 5 minutes
Cooking - 20 minutes

- 1 cal oil spray
- 1 red onion
- ½ tsp ground cinnamon
- 1 tsp ground cumin
- 350g / 12oz frozen Quorn mince
- 1 tbsp flour
- 450ml / 16 fl oz vegetable stock
- zest and juice of ½ lemon
- 410g / 14oz tin chickpeas
- bunch flat leaf parsley

Method

Chop the onion and drain and rinse the chickpeas.

Heat a large pan and fry the onion in 5 sprays of the oil for about 4-5 minutes until soft but not burnt.

Add the flour, spices and cook for a further 1 minute.

Add the stock, lemon zest and juice and the chickpeas and bring to the boil.

Add the frozen Quorn mince, bring back to a simmer and cook for 15 minutes stirring occasionally. If too thick, add a little hot water.

When ready, add the roughly chopped parsley and serve hot.

*****Quorn mince or pieces hold their texture if added to dishes frozen. Never defrost or it will go to mush.

CHILLI BEANS - 200 KCAL

This is so easy to make because it uses ready cooked beans and tomatoes. Make enough to freeze for another day.

Serves 4 - 200 calories per serving
***Suitable for freezing
Preparation - 20 minutes
Cooking - 35 minutes

- 1 cal oil spray
- 1 medium onion
- 2 garlic cloves
- 175g / 6 oz carrots
- 1 red pepper
- 1 green pepper
- 150g / 5½ oz button mushrooms
- 1 cooking apple
- 2 tbsp chilli powder
- 225g / 7½ oz chopped tomatoes
- 400g / 14 oz tin mixed beans

Method
Halve and slice the onion, crush the garlic, peel and dice the carrot, de-seed and dice both peppers.

Quarter the button mushrooms and peel, core and grate the apple.

Heat 5 sprays of the oil in a large pan and cook the onion, garlic, carrots, peppers and mushrooms for 5 minutes.

Stir in the grated apple and the chilli powder and cook for a further 2 minutes stirring well.

Add the tomatoes and mixed beans, stir well and simmer with the lid on for 30 minutes.

Make sure you keep an eye on it as it will tend to stick to the pan so stir quite often.

NOTES

LESS THAN 300 CALORIES

LEEK & BEAN FRITTATA – 215 KCAL

An easy dish to make and keeps well in the fridge and is just as delicious cold for a quick lunch for your next fasting day.

Serves 4 – 215 calories per serving
Preparation - 10 minutes
Cooking - 40 minutes

- 250g / 9oz fresh or frozen broad beans (defrosted)
- 2 leeks
- 2 courgettes/zucchini
- 1 tbsp fresh mint leaves
- 6 eggs
- 75g / 2¾ oz light mozzarella cheese

Method

Slice the leeks and wash out any soil. Thinly slice the courgettes/zucchini and chop the mint. Drain the mozzarella and cut into very small cubes.

Add the broad beans to a pan of boiling water, bring back to the boil and cook for 4 minutes.

Add the leeks and courgettes/zucchini and cook for a further 2 minutes. Drain and run under cold water to cool. Peel the outer skin from the beans and discard.

Heat a large non-stick pan and fry the vegetables with the mint for 3 minutes to remove excess water.

Beat the eggs and season with salt and freshly ground black pepper. Pour into the pan and cook gently for 5-6 minutes or until nearly set.

Meanwhile, preheat a grill to medium, sprinkle the frittata with the chopped mozzarella, brown under the grill until top is bubbling.

Slice into 8 portions and serve 2 per person with a green salad or fresh steamed broccoli.

SPINACH & MUSHROOM PIE – 220 KCAL

This is truly one of the most delicious low-calorie meals I cook. The wholegrain mustard gives it a real kick and I could eat this every day, even on my non-fasting days. It is so filling that I can't believe the calorie count.

Serves 2 – 220 calories per serving
***Suitable for freezing
Preparation - 15 minutes
Cooking - 40 minutes

- 200g / 8oz baby spinach or frozen spinach blocks
- 1 cal oil spray
- 250g / 10oz mixed small mushrooms such as chestnut / button / shitake
- 1 garlic clove
- 125ml / 4 fl oz low sodium vegetable stock
- 150g / 6oz cooked new potatoes
- 1 tbsp wholegrain mustard

- 1 tsp grated nutmeg
- 1 heaped tbsp reduced fat crème fraiche
- 2 sheets filo pastry
- 150g / 6oz each of green beans and broccoli

Method

Heat oven to 200º C / 180º C fan / Gas Mark 6

Quarter the mushrooms, crush the garlic, and cut the cooked potatoes into bite size chunks. Wilt spinach in a colander by pouring a kettle of boiling water over it.

Heat 5 sprays of the oil in a large frying pan and cook the mushrooms on a high heat until slightly browned. Add the crushed garlic and cook for another minute. Add the stock, nutmeg, mustard and potatoes, bring to the boil and simmer for a couple of minutes until reduced slightly. If using frozen spinach blocks add at this stage and cook until spinach has defrosted. Remove from the heat and season with salt and freshly ground black pepper.

Add the crème fraiche and wilted spinach and mix well. Tip into a suitable pie dish or dishes if only having one portion and allow to cool for about 5 minutes.

Lay the filo sheets onto a flat surface and spray a low cal oil spray or use oil and water spray and spread with a pastry brush.

Quarter the sheets and scrunch each piece and lay on top of the pie filling until dish is covered. If only baking one portion omit the filo pastry at this stage and freeze pie filling in a suitable container which you can defrost for another day.

Bake for 25 minutes until crispy and golden.

*****Filo pastry usually comes in packs of 10 or so. I usually unravel them and fold each sheet into small squares, put greaseproof or foil between each square to separate and freeze in a suitable container. I then just take out what I need.

*****Make sure when you are defrosting that you keep them well wrapped with foil or cling film or they will dry out and fall to pieces.

NOTES

MUSHROOM OMELETTE – 255 KCAL

Serves 1 – 255 calories
Preparation - 5-10 minutes
Cooking - 5-7 minutes

- 75g / 3 oz mushrooms
- 2 medium free-range eggs
- Handful of fresh Basil or another preferred herb
- 75g / 3 oz mixed leaf or other salad
- 5 cherry or other small tomatoes
- Dribble of olive oil and balsamic vinegar dressing

Method

Slice or chop the mushrooms and cook in a non-stick pan until soft but not shrunk too much, remove from pan and set aside.

Wipe out pan and spray with the 1 cal spray oil that you can get from most supermarkets. Lightly beat the eggs together and when pan is hot add the eggs.

Draw the eggs from the side into the middle of the pan until most of the egg liquid has gone from the top of the omelette.

Sprinkle the mushrooms on top evenly, season with salt and freshly ground pepper and when the bottom of the omelette is slightly browned, fold in half, lower heat to minimum and leave to cook very gently for about 2 minutes.

Serve with the mixed salad, tomatoes and dressing.

VEGETABLE & BEAN STEW – 260 KCAL

A warm and filling vegetable stew or hearty soup that is very quick to make.

Serves 2 - 260 calories per portion
Preparation - 10 minutes
Cooking - 20 minutes

- 1 onion
- 2 sticks celery
- 1 large leek
- 400g / 14 oz tin cannellini beans
- 500ml / 16 fl oz / 1-pint vegetable stock
- 200g / 7 oz greens (Spring greens, Sweetheart or Savoy cabbage)

Method
Split the leek in half length ways and wash under running water to remove any soil.

Roughly chop the onion, celery and leek and cook in a little oil until softened. Add the stock and drained beans and cook for about 4 minutes.

Add the greens or cabbage and cook for a further 5-8 minutes. If using Savoy Cabbage, cook until cabbage is as you like it perhaps a further 5-10 minutes according to taste.

Sprinkle with a little lemon juice and serve.

VEGGIE SAUSAGE & LENTIL PASTA - 260 KCAL

A quick and easy supper or lunch dish that is very satisfying.

Serves 1 - 246 calories per serving
Preparation - 5 minutes
Cooking - 30 minutes

- 15g / ½ oz dried Puy Lentils
- 2 vegetarian sausages
- 300ml / 10 fl oz vegetable stock
- 2 garlic cloves
- 50g button mushrooms
- 40g / 1½ oz fresh pasta

Method

Place the lentils, sliced garlic clove and stock in pan and bring to a boil. Reduce the heat, cover and simmer for 15 minutes. Cut the mushrooms in half and add to the pan after 10 minutes.

At the same time, cook the pasta according to the instructions on the pack.

Heat a grill to medium and cook the sausages until browned and cooked through or cook in the oven as directed on the packet. Cool a little and chop into largish pieces.

Drain the pasta and stir into the lentil and sausage pieces. Cook for a further 2 minutes and serve with steamed broccoli or on a bed of baby salad leaves.

SWEET POTATO CURRY WRAPS - 280 KCAL

This curry dish is very satisfying as you can have in a wrap or chapatti. This serves 4 so make sure you freeze the other portions for a quick lunch or supper.

Serves 4 – 280 calories per serving
***Suitable for freezing
Preparation - 10 minutes
Cooking - 25 minutes

- 300g / 10 oz sweet potato
- 400g / 14 oz tin Italian plum tomatoes
- 400g / 14 oz tin chickpeas
- 1 tsp dried chilli flakes
- 2 tbsp curry paste
- 100g / 4 oz baby spinach fresh or frozen
- 4 tbsp fat free yogurt or sour cream

- to serve - 1 low fat wrap or chapatti per serving

Method

Peel and cube the sweet potato and drain the chickpeas.

Cook the sweet potato for 10-12 minutes until tender. While the potato is doing cook the tomatoes, chickpeas, curry paste and chilli flakes for about 5 minutes at a gentle simmer, stirring often.

Drain the potato and add to the tomato mix. Stir in the spinach and cook until wilted or until the frozen spinach is heated through.

Warm through the chapatti as instructed for about 30 seconds, add the filling and a spoonful of the yogurt, fold in half and enjoy.

MUSHROOM RISOTTO - 284 KCAL

This risotto uses brown rice which is a great source of vitamin B. It is also lower in calories than white rice.

Serves 2 - 284 calories per serving
***Suitable for freezing
Preparation - 20 minutes
Cooking - 50 minutes

- 10g / ½ oz dried porcini mushrooms
- 225g / 8 oz mixed mushrooms
- 1 cal oil spray
- 1 small onion
- 1 garlic clove
- 125g / 4½ oz brown long grain rice
- 450ml / 16 fl oz / 1-pint vegetable stock
- 2 tbsp chopped fresh flat leaf parsley

Method

Put the dried porcini mushrooms in a bowl and pour over 150ml / ½ cup hot water. Soak for about 20 minutes or until the mushrooms have fully hydrated.

Drain but reserve the juice and add it to the stock. Roughly chop the mushrooms and finely chop the onion and garlic.

Using a large pan, sauté the mushrooms, onion and garlic in 5 sprays of the oil for about 5 minutes on a low heat, stir to avoid burning.

Add the rice to the onion mixture and stir well to coat with the oil. Add the stock, bring to a simmer, lower the heat and cook for 20 minutes or until the liquid has almost gone. Make sure you stir frequently to avoid the risotto sticking to the pan.

Cut the remaining mushrooms into quarters or smaller if using a mixture of larger mushrooms. Add to the rice and stir really well to mix in.

Cook for a further 10-15 minutes until all the liquid has been absorbed.

Check that the rice has cooked through, adding more hot water or stock if necessary. Season to taste and add the chopped parsley before serving.

BROWN RICE & VEGETABLES - 285 KCAL

This is a very easy dish to cook and you can freeze portions for a quick lunch or to accompany a main meal. Can be eaten hot or cold.

Serves 4 - 290 calories per serving
***Suitable for freezing
Preparation - 30 minutes
Cooking - 50 minutes

- 225g / 8oz dried brown rice
- 225g / 8oz carrots
- 1 onion
- 2 red peppers
- 100g / 3½ oz frozen peas
- 150g / 5½ oz mushrooms
- 2 tbsp soy sauce
- 700ml / 1¾ pints vegetable stock
- 2 tbsp tomato puree

Method

Peel and dice the carrots, chop the onion, de-seed and dice the peppers and slice the mushrooms.

Put everything except the frozen peas into a large saucepan and mix well. Bring to the boil, cover and simmer for 40 minutes, stirring occasionally to move the vegetables around.

Stir in the frozen peas and cook for a further 8 minutes or until all the liquid is gone and the rice is tender. Add more hot water if the rice is not quite cooked.

Serve with steamed broccoli.

BUTTERNUT SQUASH & PEA STEW - 285 KCAL

This dish has a lovely warming flavour because of the cinnamon and chilli powder, but it is not too spicy so give it a try.

Serves 2 - 285 calories per serving
***Suitable for freezing
Preparation - 20 minutes
Cooking - 30 minutes

- 1 tbsp lemon juice
- 1 tsp clear honey
- 1 tsp ground cinnamon
- ½ tsp chilli powder
- 1 medium onion
- 2 garlic cloves
- 375g / 12 oz butternut squash
- 60g / 2oz frozen peas
- 1 medium pitta bread to serve

Method

Halve and slice the onion and garlic. Peel the butternut squash and cut into bite size chunks.

Mix together the lemon juice, honey, cinnamon and chilli powder and leave to one side.

Cook the onion and garlic for 5 minutes in a large non-stick pan sprayed with a low-calorie cooking spray.

When the onions have started to soften add the butternut squash and the honey and lemon mixture and mix well.

Add 150ml / 5½ fl oz water, bring to the boil, lower heat and simmer for 15 minutes.

Add the peas and simmer for a further 10 minutes or until the butternut squash is ready.

Cut the pitta into slices and serve with the stew as a dip.

VEGETABLE RISOTTO – 285 KCAL

Choose your own vegetables for this risotto, whatever is in season will go well with this dish.

Serves 4 – 284 calories per serving
***Suitable for freezing
Preparation - 10 minutes
Cooking - 60 minutes

- 4 spring onions
- 250g / 9 oz dried risotto rice
- 900ml / 1½ pints hot vegetable stock
- 1 courgette/zucchini
- 2 small carrots
- 125g / 4½ oz green beans
- 100g / 3½ oz frozen peas defrosted
- 75g / 2¾ oz low fat soft cheese
- 6 fresh chives, snipped.

Method

Chop the spring onions, thinly slice the courgette/zucchini, peel and cut the carrots into matchsticks or julienne sticks and slice the beans into ½ inch pieces.

Fry the spring onions in a spray of oil in a large shallow pan or wok for 2 minutes. Add the rice and stir for a further 2 minutes until the rice appears to be opaque.

Keep the pan on a low heat and add the hot stock to the rice a ladle at a time and stir until the liquid is fully absorbed. Continue to do this until you have used about half of the stock, roughly 10 minutes. At this point add the courgette/zucchini, carrots and beans.

Carry on as before, still adding hot stock a ladle at a time and stirring until absorbed. This should take about 25-30 minutes and the rice should now be tender and creamy looking but still with a little bite but not grainy. If you run out of stock before the rice is cooked, you can use a little boiling water to top up.

Finally add the defrosted peas and heat through, then stir in the soft cheese and serve with the snipped chives on top.

FIVE BEAN WRAP - 294 KCAL

This is a very filling meal and can be eaten for lunch or dinner depending on your schedule. Most food shops now stock many different types of ready cooked beans in either cans or pouches. Try a tin of the mixed bean salad variety which lends itself very well to this recipe.

Serves 1 - 294 calories per serving
Preparation 5 minutes

- 1 reduced calorie wrap
- 80g / 3oz ready-to-eat mixed beans
- 20g / ¾ oz low calorie or lighter cheddar cheese
- 1 tbsp any salsa
- shredded lettuce

Method
Rinse and drain the beans. Spread your chosen salsa evenly over the whole wrap.

Add the drained beans but leave at least two inches/5cm free at the bottom of the wrap so that you can fold it over easier.

Put the lettuce on top of the beans and finally grate the cheese evenly over the lettuce. Fold up the bottom of the wrap and roll up the rest. You may wish to warm the wrap up a bit first as it will be easier to roll but this is not essential.

HEARTY SUMMER SALAD - 294 KCAL

This recipe serves 3 because you are using canned beans. It will keep in the fridge if you want to just use 1 or 2 portions or if you can get smaller tins of beans then adjust accordingly. Use medium tomatoes instead of large and half a medium onion. Everything else is fine as it is.

Serves 3 - 294 calories a portion
Preparation - 5-10 minutes

- 400g / 14 oz. can chickpeas
- 400g / 14 oz. can cannellini Beans
- 300g / 11 oz jar artichoke hearts
- 2 large tomatoes
- ½ large onion
- 3 large fresh garlic cloves
- dribble olive oil and balsamic vinegar
- a few pinches of dried parsley
- fresh ground salt and pepper to taste
- 150g / 5 oz mixed salad leaves

Method

Drain chickpeas and cannellini beans and put them into a large bowl. Chop artichoke hearts (into eighths if they're whole, or into quarters if they're already halved) and add to bowl.

Chop the tomatoes, dice the onion and crush garlic gloves and add these also to the bowl.

Whip olive oil and balsamic vinegar together, and then pour over the pile in the bowl. Add a few generous pinches of dried parsley, then salt and pepper to taste.

Stir all the ingredients thoroughly with a large spoon to distribute them evenly and coat them with vinaigrette. Serve on a bed of mixed salad.

NUTTY MUSHROOM PILAF – 298 KCAL

Using Bulgar wheat instead of brown rice for a delicious nutty flavour makes this dish low in calories. You can also use dried porcini or other mixed mushrooms instead.

Serves 2 – 298 calories per serving
Preparation - 5 minutes
Cooking - 30 minutes

- 4 large flat mushrooms
- 1 onion
- 2 garlic cloves
- 110g / 4 oz dried bulgar wheat
- 600ml / 20 fl oz vegetable stock
- 50g / 1¾ oz broccoli florets
- 3 tbsp low fat soft cheese
- 2 tbsp chopped dill

Method

Slice the mushrooms and garlic and cut the onion into wedges.

Heat a non-stick frying pan until hot and spray with the cooking oil. Fry the onion and mushrooms for 5 minutes, add the garlic and cook for another 2 minutes.

Add the bulgar wheat to the pan together with the stock and bring to a simmer. Cover and cook for 5 minutes.

Add the broccoli and cook for a further 5 minutes or until the bulgar wheat is cooked and the stock has been absorbed. If not quite cooked, add a little more hot water.

Stir in the chopped dill and soft cheese and season to taste.

NOTES

LESS THAN 400 CALORIES

VEGETABLE STEW & DUMPLINGS - 315 KCAL

You can use any seasonal or favourite vegetables for this dish. The dumplings give it a really satisfying feeling.

Serves 4 - 315 calories per serving
***Suitable for freezing
Preparation - 35 minutes
Cooking - 45 minutes

- 1 cal oil spray
- 90g / 3¼ oz shallots or small onions
- 1 medium leek
- 225g / 8 oz parsnips
- 1 large carrot
- 1.2 ltr / 2 pints vegetable stock
- 25g / 1oz bulgar wheat
- 400g tin cannellini beans
- 150g / 5 oz small cauliflower florets
- handful of chopped parsley
- 90g / 3¼ oz self-raising flour
- 1 tsp ground coriander
- 1 tsp cumin seeds
- 2 tbsp low fat spread

Method

Halve the shallots or small onions, slice and thoroughly wash the leek, peel and slice the carrot and peel and chop the parsnips.

Make the dumplings by sifting the flour and cumin powder into a large bowl. Add the cumin seeds and rub in the low-fat spread until all combined. Add a small amount of water, just enough to make a soft dough. Make into 8 dumplings and set aside.

Heat 5 sprays of the oil in a large saucepan and fry the onions, leek, carrot and parsnip for about 6 minutes until soft but not browned.

Add the stock, bulgar wheat and beans and bring to the boil. Reduce heat, cover pan and simmer for 20 minutes.

Add the cauliflower and stir, then place the dumplings on top of the stew, cover and simmer gently for a further 20 minutes or until the dumplings are cooked through.

Season to taste and sprinkle over the parsley. Serve or freeze at this point giving 2 dumplings to each portion.

PASTA & CHERRY TOMATOES - 325 KCAL

A low-fat recipe that is quite filling as well as being tasty and very quick and easy to make

Serves 1 - 325 calories
Preparation - 5 minutes
Cooking - 15 minutes

- 100g / 4 oz cherry tomatoes
- 3 black olives
- 1 clove of garlic, peeled
- A handful of basil
- 1 cal oil spray
- 75g / 3 oz fresh pasta
- Salt and black pepper
- bag mixed salad leaves or rocket

Method
Chop the tomatoes, olives and garlic. Put them into a bowl with some basil, then drizzle with the oil and stir well.

Cook the pasta as directed usually 4 minutes for fresh pasta.

Once the pasta is cooked, drain and rinse through with boiling water and return to the pan.

Add the tomato mixture from the bowl and stir over a very low heat. Add salt and black pepper and serve immediately with a big helping of mixed salad leaves.

SWEETCORN SOUFFLé - 325 KCAL

Don't be nervous about cooking a soufflé you will be surprised how easy they are to make, and this dish has only a few ingredients.

Serves 2 - 284 calories per serving
Preparation - 12 minutes
Cooking - 60 minutes

- 2 eggs
- 25g / 1 oz plain flour
- 200ml / 7 fl oz skimmed milk
- 200g / 7oz tin sweetcorn
- 60g / 2oz half fat cheddar cheese
- ½ green pepper

Method

Preheat the oven to 180°C / 160° C fan / Gas 4

Very lightly oil a 700ml / 1¼ pint soufflé dish or 2 smaller individual dishes. (or use a low-calorie spray).

Whisk together the eggs and flour and then slowly whisk in the milk a little at a time. When combined, stir in the drained sweetcorn, grated cheese and de-seeded and chopped green pepper. Season to taste.

Pour mixture into the prepared soufflé dish or individual dishes and bake for 1 hour until puffed up and nicely browned but not burnt. The smaller dishes will only take about 45 minutes.

Serve with steamed broccoli and courgettes/zucchini.

LEEK & MUSHROOM BAKE – 330 KCAL

Serves 2 – 330 calories per serving
Preparation - 20 minutes
Cooking - 50 minutes

- 6 medium open mushrooms
- 2 garlic cloves
- 2 medium leeks
- 400g / 14 oz tin chopped tomatoes
- 1 tsp mixed dried herbs
- 1 tbsp tomato puree

For the crumble
- 50g / 1¾ oz plain white flour
- 25g / 1 oz porridge oats
- ½ tsp English mustard powder
- 15g / ½ oz low fat spread
- 50g / 1¾ oz half fat Cheddar cheese

Method
Preheat the oven to 190º / 170º C fan / Gas 5

Halve and thickly slice the mushrooms and the leeks.

Peel and crush the garlic. Stir fry the mushrooms and leeks for 5 minutes in an oiled frying pan.

Add the garlic and cook for a further 2 minutes. Add the tomatoes, tomato puree, herbs and seasoning and simmer for 10 minutes.

For the topping, mix together the flour, oats, mustard powder and low-fat spread and rub together until it resembles breadcrumbs.

Add the cheese and season to taste. Place the mushroom and leek mixture in an oven proof casserole dish and cover with the crumb mixture.

Cook in the oven for about 30 minutes or until the crumble is crisp and browned.

Serve with a big portion of steamed broccoli.

MIXED VEGETABLE BAKE – 330 KCAL

This is a substantial vegetable dish with a potato and cheese topping. This is unusual for a low-calorie meal so enjoy it. You can also make individual portions for the freezer.

Serves 4 – 330 calories per serving
***Suitable for freezing
Preparation – 10 minutes
Cooking – 25-30 minutes

- 2 medium onions
- 1 garlic clove
- 2 peppers, 1 red and 1 green
- 1 medium aubergine/egg plant
- 2 medium courgettes/zucchini
- 2 x 400g /14oz tins chopped tomatoes
- ½ tbsp dried mixed herbs
- 2 tbsp tomato puree
- 900g / 2lb potatoes
- 75g / 2¾ oz grated low fat cheese

Method
Finely chop the onions and garlic.

Deseed and halve and slice the peppers. Top and tail the aubergine/eggplant and cut into small chunks. Trim and thinly slice the courgettes/zucchini.

Put the onion, garlic, peppers, dried herbs, tomato puree and the 2 tins of chopped tomatoes in a large pan. Bring to the boil, cover and simmer gently for 10 minutes, stirring occasionally.

Stir in the aubergine/eggplant and courgettes/zucchini and cook uncovered for another 10 minutes, giving it the occasional stir.

While the vegetables are cooking, peel and cut the potatoes into 2.5cm / 1-inch pieces. Boil them for 7-10 minutes until cooked through and then drain.

Put the vegetables into ovenproof dishes, depending on your chosen portion size. Place the potatoes on top of the vegetable mixture, dividing equally if using smaller dishes. Sprinkle the cheese on top of the potatoes.

Freeze your other portions at this stage.

Preheat your grill to medium and grill the dish for 5 minutes until the cheese is bubbling and the potatoes are getting golden and crispy. Serve on warmed plates with nothing else.

VEGETARIAN SHEPHERD'S PIE - 340 KCAL

A tasty meat free traditional shepherd's pie that is very satisfying on a cold winter's day. Can be frozen in individual portions.

Serves 4 - 340 calories per serving
***Suitable for freezing
Preparation - 40 minutes
Cooking - 50 minutes

- 500g / 1lb 2oz sweet potato
- 1 onion
- 3 garlic cloves
- 1 celery stick
- 2 carrots
- 1 tbsp chopped tarragon
- 350g / 14oz pack frozen Quorn mince
- 1 tbsp flour
- 700g jar passata
- 400g / 14 oz tin cannellini beans
- 25g / 1oz half fat grated cheese
- 50g / 2oz frozen peas and sweetcorn mix

Method

Peel the sweet potato and cut into chunks. Finely chop the onion and crush the garlic cloves. Peel and finely dice the celery and carrots.

Boil the sweet potato for 15 minutes or until tender. Drain and mash with seasoning to taste.

Fry the onion, carrot, celery and garlic in a large non-stick saucepan for 5 minutes. Add the chopped tarragon and cook for a further 5 minutes. Add the flour and stir, pour in the passata and bring back to the boil.

Add the frozen mince, peas and sweetcorn and the cannellini beans and heat gently until bubbling. Remove from the heat and season well.

Divide mixture into relevant portions and top each one with the mash. Sprinkle over the cheese and bake in a preheated oven 190ºC / 375ºF / Gas 5 for 40-45 minutes depending on portion size, or until golden brown.

You can either defrost and cook for 40-45 minutes or from frozen for 50-55 minutes at the same temperatures.

VEGETABLE & QUORN STEW - 345 KCAL

This is a really lovely stew with a deep rich flavour. Make a bigger batch and freeze portions for another day, well worth the effort.

Serves 2 – 355 calories per serving
***Suitable for freezing
Preparation - 10 minutes
Cooking - 50 minutes

- 1 cal oil spray
- 1 onion
- 200g / 7 oz Quorn pieces
- 50g / 2 oz dried apricots
- 30g / 1 oz sun-dried tomatoes
- 400g / 14oz tin chopped tomatoes
- 400g / 14 oz potatoes
- 1 tsp dried basil
- 1 vegetable stock cube
- 200ml / 7 fl oz water

Method

Chop the onion and apricots, slice the sun-dried tomatoes and peel and cut the potatoes into chunks.

Heat 5 sprays of the oil in a large pan and fry the onion for 5 minutes until soft. Add the Quorn pieces, apricots, sun-dried and canned tomatoes with the water and bring to a boil.

Crumble in the stock cube, turn down the heat and simmer for 20 minutes, stirring occasionally until nice and thick. Season to taste.

In the meantime, boil the potato chunks for about 10 minutes, depending on size, drain and add to the stew.

Cook for a further 5 minutes and serve.

LOW FAT PESTO TAGLIATELLE - 350 KCAL

Pesto sauce is quite high in fat content, but this homemade sauce uses fromage frais instead of oil and is therefore much healthier. You can also use any colour pasta you like or try a combination of green and white tagliatelle.

Serves 2 - 350 calories per portion
***Suitable for freezing
Preparation - 10 minutes
Cooking - 15 minutes

- 125g / 4½ oz chestnut or other mixed mushrooms
- 75ml / 3 oz / ⅓ cup vegetable stock
- 90g / 3½ oz asparagus
- 150g / 5 oz fresh tagliatelle
- 200g / 7 oz ready to eat artichoke hearts
- Parmesan shavings

Pesto sauce
- 1 garlic clove
- 15g / ½ oz fresh basil leaves

- 3 tbsp low-fat natural fromage frais
- 1 tbsp grated Parmesan cheese
- salt & pepper

Method

Make the pesto sauce by either using a blender or finely chopping the basil and mixing it well with all the other ingredients.

To make the pasta, slice the mushrooms, place in a small pan with the stock, bring to the boil and poach in the vegetable stock for 4 minutes. Drain and set aside.

Rinse out the pan, trim and cut the asparagus into 5cm (2") lengths and cook in boiling water for 3-4 minutes, drain and set aside.

Cook the pasta as directed on the packet, drain, sprinkle with a little olive oil to stop it sticking, return to the pan. Add the mushrooms, cooked asparagus, and the drained and halved artichoke hearts and cook on a very low heat for about 2 minutes.

Remove from heat and stir in the pesto sauce and serve with a few shredded basil leaves and the parmesan shavings.

VEGETARIAN POTATO CURRY - 350 KCAL

This is a very easy one-pot meal that you will cook again and again just because it is so delicious and quick to do. You will even consider having it on your non-fasting days with rice and a naan.

serves 2 - 350 calories per serving
***Suitable for freezing
Preparation - 10 minutes
Cooking - 30 minutes

- 100g / 4 oz red lentils
- 450ml / 15 fl oz / 1¾ cups vegetable stock
- 1 small onion
- 2 medium tomatoes
- 1 tsp turmeric
- 1 tsp garam masala
- 1 red chilli
- 1 large sweet potato
- 2 handfuls baby spinach

Method

Finely chop the onion and chilli. Roughly chop the tomatoes. Peel and cube the sweet potato and shred the baby spinach.

Put the lentils, stock, onion, tomatoes, spices and the red chilli into a pan, bring to a simmer and cook for 10 minutes. Add the sweet potato and cook for a further 10 minutes or until done.

Stir in the shredded baby spinach and season to taste. When spinach is wilted, serve at once.

BUTTERNUT SQUASH RISOTTO – 365 KCAL

Risotto is a very easy dish to master once you get the hang of it. This recipe serves 4 but it freezes well so you can have some more ready meals in the freezer.

Serves 2 – 365 calories per serving
***Suitable for freezing
Preparation – 10 minutes
Cooking – 20-25 minutes

- 1 small onion
- 1 cal oil spray
- 1 x 250g / 9 oz butternut squash
- 150g / 5 oz carnnaroli or arborio risotto rice
- 600ml / 1¼ pint / 2½ cups vegetable stock
- 2 tbsp grated parmesan

Method

Chop the onion finely. Peel and dice the butternut squash or pumpkin.

Heat 10 sprays of the oil in a large pan and fry the onion until softened.

Add the rice and stir until coated in the oil. Add the squash and half the hot stock and stir well. Cook, stirring often until most of the stock has been absorbed.

Then add a little stock at a time, again stirring until absorbed.

Repeat this until all the stock has been used and the rice and squash are cooked. The rice should have a little bite but not grainy. Add more stock or hot water if needed.

Add the cheese to the rice and stir well. Cover the pan and leave to sit for 1 minute.

Season well and dish out into warmed bowls. Add a very tiny splash of olive oil to each bowl and serve.

GOLDEN RICE & ONIONS - 365 KCAL

This dish has a hint of Indian spices and the turmeric gives the rice a warming yellow colour. Leave the onion out or use plain onions if not to your taste but they do add a little more colour and flavour.

Serves 2 - 365 per portion
***Suitable for freezing
Preparation - 10 minutes
Cooking - 25-30 minutes

- 90g / 3½ oz basmati rice
- 30g / 1 oz red lentils
- 1 bay leaf
- 3 cardamom pods, split
- 1 tsp ground turmeric
- 3 cloves
- ½ tsp cumin seeds
- ½ cinnamon stick
- 1 small onion
- 125g / 4½ oz cauliflower florets
- 1 medium carrot
- 50g / 2 oz frozen peas

- 30g / 1 oz sultanas
- 300ml / 10 fl oz / 1¼ cups vegetable stock
- salt & pepper
- 1 tbsp chopped fresh coriander (optional)

For the Onions
- 1 cal oil spray
- 1 small red onion
- 1 small white onion
- 1 tsp caster sugar

Method

Peel and dice the carrot, break the cauliflower into small florets. Put the carrot, cauliflower, onion, rice, lentils, spices, bay leaf, peas and sultanas into a large pan. Season and thoroughly mix.

Pour over the stock, bring to the boil, cover and simmer for 15 minutes stirring occasionally to avoid the rice sticking. Add more stock if it runs dry before the rice is cooked.

When the rice is tender, remove, cover and it let stand for about 10 minutes or until all the liquid has been absorbed.

Take out the bay leaf, cardamom pods, cloves and cinnamon stick.

While the rice is cooking, shred the onions, heat the 5 sprays of the oil in a frying pan and fry the onions over a medium heat for 4 minutes until just starting to soften.

Add the sugar, turn up the heat and cook, stirring all the time for a further 2-3 minutes until golden but not burnt.

Stir the rice mixture through and serve on warmed plates with the onions on top and sprinkled with the chopped coriander if liked.

NOTES

MUSHROOM RISOTTO - 365 KCAL

I have included a higher calorie mushroom risotto because not everyone likes brown rice. You can use any variety of mushrooms you like.

Serves 1 - 365 calories
***Suitable for freezing
Preparation - 5-10 minutes
Cooking - 20-25 minutes

- 1 small onion
- 125g / 4½ oz mixed mushrooms
- 1 cal oil spray
- 80g / 3 oz risotto rice
- 250ml / 8 fl oz / 1 cup of hot vegetable stock
- 20g / 1 oz Parmesan cheese, grated
- A small handful of flat leaved parsley, chopped

Method

Chop the onions and garlic and wipe the mushrooms before also chopping them.

Warm the oil in a large pan, add the onions and garlic and cook gently for 2 minutes. Then add the mixed mushrooms and cook for another minute or so.

Add the risotto rice and stir well to coat the rice with the juices for about a minute. Add enough of the hot stock to cover the rice and cook, stirring constantly until the liquid has been absorbed.

Add more hot stock and continue to stir as this is also absorbed, (for best results you should keep the stock hot in a separate pan on the stove).

Repeat this process, stirring as you do, until the rice is ready, there should be a hint of grain but not too hard. Add more boiling water if necessary when stock has been used up.

Remove from heat, stir in the Parmesan and chopped parsley, check the seasoning and allow to stand for 1 minute before serving on warmed plates.

PENNE & PEPPER SAUCE - 375 KCAL

Pasta makes a filling supper dish but don't have it too often. However, because this only uses vegetables it is also very healthy.

Serves 2 - 375 calories
***Suitable for freezing
Preparation - 15 minutes
Cooking - 20 minutes

- 1 red and 1 yellow pepper
- 1 medium red onion
- 2 cloves of garlic
- 1 cal oil spray
- 175g / 6 oz fresh penne pasta
- salt and black pepper

Method

Halve the peppers and remove the seeds and membranes. Rub the skins with a few sprays of oil and place them, skin sides up, on a piece of foil under a hot grill.

Once the skins have burnt and turned brown, remove from grill and allow cool slightly. Pull off the skin, slice and put into a small mixing bowl.

Chop the onion and garlic. Cook the pasta as directed on the pack. While the pasta is cooking, put 5 sprays of the oil in a large frying pan and gently fry the onion and garlic.

Add the peppers and juices from the bowl and continue cooking, stirring them together. Add some pasta liquid to keep the sauce moist if necessary. When the pasta is cooked, drain and return it to the pan.

Add the pepper sauce, salt and lots of black pepper. Stir thoroughly and serve.

BAKED VEGGIE BOLOGNESE - 385 KCAL

This dish is so easy to make and is absolutely delicious. Even though it is for 4 you really should make and freeze the remainder because you will be eating it often.

Serves 4 - 380 calories per serving
***Suitable for freezing
Preparation - 15 minutes
Cooking - 40 - 50 minutes

- 1 small onion
- 2 garlic cloves
- 350g / 12 oz packet Quorn or vegetarian mince
- 400g / 14 oz tin chopped tomatoes
- 1 tbsp dried oregano
- 1 tsp mixed dried herbs
- 1 tbsp tomato puree
- 150 ml / 5 fl oz vegetable stock
- 125g / 4½ oz fresh fusilli or other small pasta shapes
- 300g / 10½ oz low fat soft cheese
- 2 egg yolks

Method

Preheat the oven to 180º C / 160º C fan / Gas 4

Grate the onion and crush the garlic.

In a large bowl mix together the onion, garlic, mince, tomatoes, oregano and tomato puree. Stir the stock into the mixture and add the fresh pasta, season well. Turn into a 1½ litre / 2¾ pint oven-proof dish. Mix the soft cheese and egg yolks together and season well. Spread over the top of the mince mixture and bake in the oven for 40-45 minutes. Serve with a good portion of steamed broccoli.

TOFU & NOODLES - 386 KCAL

Tofu is very low in fat and will absorb flavours if you marinate it long enough. Just make sure you cook with plenty of spices and herbs

Serves 2 - 385 calories per serving
Preparation - 10 minutes + 1-hour marinating
Cooking - 15 minutes

- 100g / 3½ oz firm tofu
- 1 tbsp light soy sauce
- 2½ cm / 1-inch piece fresh ginger
- 2 garlic cloves
- 40g / 1½ oz dried egg noodles
- 150g / 5½oz frozen spinach
- 2 spring onions or scallions
- 1 tsp sesame seeds
- ½ tsp dried chilli flakes

Method
Drain and cube the tofu, peel and finely grate the ginger, crush the garlic, chop the frozen spinach and the spring onions.

Marinate the Tofu by placing in a small bowl and adding the soy sauce, ginger and garlic and mix together. Leave for about an hour if possible.

When Tofu is ready, cook the noodles in a large pan according to the packet instructions until soft.

Lightly oil a wok or large frying pan and add the spinach and spring onions and stir fry for a couple of minutes until tender and thoroughly defrosted if using frozen spinach.

Add the tofu and marinade to the pan, toss in the noodles, sesame oil and seeds and turn gently until the tofu is heated through. Sprinkle over the chilli flakes and some coriander or parsley if liked.

MUSHROOMS & MUSTARD MASH - 390 KCAL

Mushrooms are a filling and tasty main dish and when served with this polenta mash you will have a substantial evening meal.

Serves 2 - 390 calories per serving
Preparation - 10 minutes
Cooking - 15 minutes

- 600ml / 20 fl oz vegetable stock
- 1 tsp corn flour
- 1 small onion
- 2 garlic cloves
- 250g / 9 oz chestnut mushrooms
- 125ml / 4 fl oz red wine
- 2 tbsp cranberry sauce
- 100g / 3½ oz dried quick cook Polenta
- 2 tsp wholegrain mustard
- 30g / 1¼ oz grated mature cheese

Method
Finely chop the onion, crush the garlic and thickly slice the mushrooms.

Bring 400ml / 14 fl oz of the vegetable stock to the boil and blend the corn flour with the remaining 200ml / 6 fl oz.

Spray a non-stick pan with oil and fry the garlic, onions and mushrooms for about 5 minutes. Add the red wine and cook for a further minute. Slowly add the remaining corn flour stock and the cranberry sauce.

Cook gently for 2 minutes until nice and thick, season to taste and remove from heat and keep warm.

Once the stock is boiling, slowly add the Polenta, stir and cook for 1-2 minutes until thickened.

Stir in the mustard and cheese and serve straight away with the mushrooms and sauce.

VEGETARIAN CHILLI - 390 KCAL

This is high in calories because of the rice. If you want to eat it without the rice, then the calorie count drops to only 125 calories for the chilli alone. You could eat it with a green salad or for a more substantial meal try having it in a flatbread with some lettuce which will only add up to 225 calories.

Serves 2 - 390 per serving
***Suitable for freezing
Preparation - 5 minutes
Cooking - 20 minutes

- 1 red chilli
- 200g / 7 oz mushrooms
- 1 garlic clove
- 1 tsp cumin
- 400g / 14 oz can chopped tomatoes
- 400g / 14 oz can red kidney beans

To serve

- 150g / 5 oz cooked brown rice

Method

Fry the finely chopped garlic and red chilli in 1 tbsp of olive oil with the cumin.

Add the chopped mushrooms and cook for about 4 minutes more but add some water if the mushrooms do not release enough liquid.

Add the chopped tomatoes and kidney beans, stir and cook for another 10 minutes on a very low heat making sure you stir often, or it will stick. Serve with the cooked brown rice.

COURGETTE & CHEESE TART - 398 KCAL

This is so simple to make because you can use ready rolled puff pastry if you want and that's about as hard as it gets. It is not suitable for freezing but will keep in the fridge for a few days so have a slice for lunch or share it with the family.

Serves 2 - 398 calories per serving
Preparation - 10 minutes
Cooking - 50 minutes

- 125g / 4½ oz ready rolled puff pastry
- 110g / 4 oz Brie cheese
- 2 large ripe tomatoes
- 110g / 4 oz courgettes/zucchini
- ½ tsp dried oregano

Method
Pre-heat oven to 200°C / 375 F / Gas 6

Roll out the pastry to a 12 x 15 cm / 4½ inch x 6-inch oblong and put on a damp baking sheet.

Mark the pastry all around the edge with a sharp knife 2.5cm / 1 inch from the edge. Prick the centre space within the marks with a fork.

Slice the Brie, tomatoes and courgettes/zucchini into fairly thin slices. Heat a tbsp of olive oil in a small frying pan and fry the courgettes/zucchini for about 2 minutes until softened and then add the oregano and cook for a further 1 minute.

Set aside to cool enough to handle.

Starting at one of the smaller ends, make rows of the brie, courgette/zucchini and tomatoes slices within the centre oblong overlapping each layer.

Drizzle over any pan juices left and bake for 20-25 minutes or until the pastry is nicely risen and golden brown.

Serve with a green salad or steamed broccoli.

NOTES

CALORIE COUNTER

All calories given are for 100g or 100ml liquids

BEANS & LENTILS
Baked beans -- 83
Black Eye beans -- 455
Butter beans -- 270
Chickpeas -- 320
Flageolet beans -- 279
Haricot -- 69
Lentils (brown) -- 297
Lentils (green) -- 316
Lentils (red) -- 327
Lentils (yellow) -- 334
Lima butter beans -- 282
Pinto beans -- 309
Puy lentils -- 307

Red kidney beans -- 311
Soybeans -- 375
White beans -- 285

BREADS
Baguette -- 242
Chapatti -- 278
Ciabatta -- 269
Gluten-free -- 282
Pita, white -- 265
Pumpernickel -- 183
Rye -- 242
Soda, brown -- 223
Sourdough -- 256
Spelt -- 241
Whole grain -- 260
Whole wheat -- 234
Bagels -- 256
Plain croissant -- 414
Crumpets -- 180

BREAKFAST CEREALS
All bran -- 334
Alpen -- 361
Dorset cereal muesli -- 356
Granola -- 432
Kallo milk choc rice cakes -- 495
Muesli (unsweetened) -- 353
Oatmeal -- 363

Porridge Oats -- 355
Porridge (ready to eat) per serving -- 95
Oat So Simple instant porridge -- 380
Special K -- 379

CAKES
Apple pie -- 262
Apple tart -- 265
Baklava -- 498
Brownies -- 419
Carrot cake, iced -- 359
Chewing gum, sugar-free -- 159
Chocolate (dark) -- 547
Chocolate (milk) -- 549
Chocolate (white) -- 567
Chocolate cake, iced -- 414
Chocolate chip cookies -- 499
Chocolate croissant -- 433
Chocolate mousse -- 174
Chocolate-covered raisins -- 418
Cinnamon buns -- 280
Crystallized ginger -- 351
Digestives Mcvities -- 478
Flapjacks, all-butter -- 457
Ice cream, vanilla -- 190
Lemon cake -- 366
Liquorice -- 325
Marshmallow -- 338
Meringue -- 394

Mince pies -- 398
Oatmeal raisin cookies -- 445
Pain aux raisins -- 335
Peppermints -- 395
Scones -- 366
Sherbet, lemon -- 390
Shortbread, all-butter -- 523
Sorbet, lemon -- 118
Tiramisu -- 263
Toffee -- 459
Yoghurt-covered dried fruit -- 447

CHEESE
Babybel -- 362
Babybel light -- 210
Boursin -- 405
Boursin light -- 140
Brie -- 320
Camembert -- 290
Cheddar cheese (low-fat) -- 263
Cheddar, mature, medium -- 410
Cottage cheese (low-fat) -- 72
Cottage cheese, plain -- 101
Cream cheese (low-fat) -- 109
Danish blue -- 342
Dolcelatte -- 395
Edam -- 341
Emmenthal -- 370
Feta -- 250

Goat cheese, soft -- 324
Gouda -- 377
gruyere -- 396
Parmesan cheese (fresh, grated) -- 389
Philadelphia cream cheese (low-fat) -- 111
Philadelphia cream cheese (normal) -- 245
Ricotta -- 134
Roquefort -- 368

DRIED FRUIT
Açai (dried berry powder) 1G -- 5
Cherries (glacé) -- 313
Dried apple -- 310
Dried apricot -- 196
Dried banana chips -- 523
Dried blueberries -- 313
Dried cranberries -- 346
Dried dates (pitted) -- 303
Dried figs -- 229
Dried mango -- 268
Dried prunes -- 151
Raisins -- 292

DRINKS
Apple juice -- 44
Beer, bitter -- 32
Beer, lager -- 43
Cappuccino, whole milk -- 37
Cappuccino, skimmed milk -- 22

Champagne -- 76
Coca cola -- 43
Coffee (black) -- 0
Coffee (with semi-skimmed milk) -- 7
Coke (diet) -- 0
Coke (normal) -- 43
Cordial (elderflower) -- 27
Cordial (lime) -- 24
Espresso -- 20
Gin and tonic -- 70
Ginger ale (dry) -- 34
Hot chocolate -- 59
Hot chocolate (low-cal) -- 19
Hot milk and honey (semi-sk) -- 58
Innocent smoothie (mango) -- 56
Innocent smoothie (straw/banana) --53
Latte (skimmed milk) -- 29
Latte (whole milk) -- 54
Lemonade -- 47
Lime juice -- 23
Macchiato (skimmed milk) -- 26
Macchiato (whole milk) -- 30
Milkshakes (strawberry) -- 67
Orange juice -- 42
Orange squash -- 10
Pear juice -- 43
Red wine -- 68
Ribena -- 43

Sparkling water -- 0
Sprite -- 44
Tea (black) -- 0
Tea (chai latte, semi-skimmed milk) -- 70
Tea (green) (herbal) -- 0
Vodka tonic -- 71
Wheatgrass (frozen juice) -- 17
White wine -- 66

EGGS
Egg whites -- 50
Eggs (fried) -- 187
Eggs (omelette) -- 173
Eggs (poached) -- 145
Eggs (scrambled) -- 155
Eggs (boiled) -- 147

I have included the calorie counter for Fish as some people are just non-meat eaters rather than fully Vegetarian.

FISH & SEAFOOD
Anchovies, canned in oil, drained -- 191
Calamari (battered, frozen) -- 200
Cod steaks, grilled -- 95
Crab, boiled -- 128
Dover sole -- 78
Eels, jellied -- 98
Fish, unbreaded -- 76

Haddock (fillets) -- 74
Halibut -- 100
Herring, raw or grilled -- 190
Kipper fillets, smoked -- 198
Kippers, grilled -- 255
Lemon sole, steamed -- 91
Mackerel (fillets) -- 204
Mussels -- 92
Plaice, steamed -- 93
Prawns, boiled -- 99
Prawns, king, cooked & peeled -- 76
Salmon (canned) -- 131
Salmon, fillet, grilled -- 169
Sardines (fresh) -- 165
Sardines (tinned, in water) -- 179
Scallops -- 83
Sea bass (fillets) -- 133
Seafood (unbreaded) -- 76
Sushi -- 156
Tuna (canned) -- 108
Tuna (fresh) -- 137

FRUIT
Apples -- 51
Apricots -- 32
Bananas -- 103
Blackberries -- 26
Blueberries -- 60
Cherries -- 52

Clementines -- 41
Compote (apple & blackberry) -- 107
Cranberries -- 42
Figs -- 230
Goji berries -- 313
Grapefruit -- 30
Grapes -- 66
Kiwi -- 55
Lemon -- 20
Limes -- 12
Mandarin -- 35
Melon -- 29
Nectarines -- 44
Oranges -- 40
Papaya -- 40
Peaches -- 37
Pears -- 41
Pineapple -- 43
Plums -- 39
Pomegranate -- 55
Prunes (tinned) -- 90
Raspberries -- 30
Satsumas -- 31
Smoothies (strawberry/banana) -- 51
Strawberries -- 28
Tangerines -- 39
Watermelon -- 33

GRAINS
Barley -- 364
Buckwheat -- 343
Buckwheat noodles -- 363
Bulgar -- 334
Corn (popping) -- 339
Cous cous -- 358
Cream crackers -- 437
Matzo crackers -- 381
Millet -- 354
Noodles (instant) -- 450
Oats -- 369
Oat cakes -- 440
Ryvita (original) -- 350
Quinoa -- 375
Ramen noodles -- 361

RICE
Arborio rice -- 354
Basmati -- 350
Brown rice -- 340
Jasmine -- 352
Long grain -- 355
Paella -- 349
Short grain -- 351
Uncle Ben's white rice (long grain) -- 344
Wild rice -- 353

Rice cakes -- 379
Rice noodles -- 373
Rye -- 331
Spelt -- 314
Tortilla -- 307
Vermicelli noodles -- 354
Wheat berries -- 326
Whole grain cereal -- 345
Whole grain pasta -- 326
Whole wheat cereal -- 359
Whole wheat pasta -- 326

HERBS & SPICES – all 1g
Basil -- 0
Cinnamon -- 3
Cloves -- 3
Coriander -- 0
Cumin -- 4
Ginger -- 1
Lemongrass -- 1
Mint -- 0
Nutmeg -- 4
Oregano -- 3
Paprika -- 3
Parsley -- 0
Pepper -- 3
Rosemary -- 0
Saffron -- 3
Sage -- 3

Tamarind paste -- 1.5
Tarragon -- 0
Thyme -- 2
Turmeric -- 3

MILK & CREAM
per 100g or 100ml liquid

Almond milk -- 24
Goats milk (whole) -- 61
Greek yoghurt -- 132
Milk (whole) -- 64
Milk (semi skimmed) -- 50
Milk (1%) -- 41
Milk (skim) -- 35
Rice milk -- 46
Soy milk -- 42

Clotted cream -- 586
Crème fraiche (low-fat) -- 79
Crème fraiche (normal) -- 299
Custard -- 118
Double Cream -- 496
Fromage frais -- 105
Fruit yoghurt -- 94
Single Cream -- 193
Sour cream (low-fat) -- 104
Sour cream (normal) -- 192
Whipped cream -- 368

Yoghurt
(low-fat, with active cultures) -- 66

NUTS
Almond (ground) -- 618
Almonds (flaked) -- 641
Almonds (whole) -- 613
Brazils -- 680
Cashews -- 583
Hazelnuts -- 660
Macadamias -- 748
Nuts (mixed, unsalted) -- 661
Peanuts -- 561
Pecans -- 698
Pine nuts -- 688
Pistachio -- 584
Walnuts -- 703

OILS & FATS
per 100g or 100ml liquid

Butter (unsalted) -- 739
Butter (salted) -- 739
Corn oil -- 829
Flaxseed oil -- 813
Flora -- 410
Hemp oil -- 837
Lard -- 899
Margarine -- 735

Olive oil -- 823
Olive oil spread -- 543
Rapeseed oil -- 825
Sunflower oil -- 828
Vegetable oil -- 827

PICKLES
Black olives (pitted, drained) -- 154
Capers -- 32
Chutney, tomato -- 141
Cornichons -- 34
Gherkins -- 38
Jalapeño -- 18
Piccalilli sauce -- 80
Pickled onions -- 36

SANDWICHES
Cheese and chutney -- 228
Egg and cress -- 232
Ham and cheese -- 288
Tuna salad -- 221

**SAUCES/DIPS/DRESSINGS
per 100g or 100ml liquid**

Savoury
Barbecue sauce -- 144
Béarnaise sauce -- 580
Bolognaise sauce (no meat) -- 50

Gravy (vege, readymade) -- 45
Heinz salad cream -- 333
Hollandaise sauce -- 239
HP brown sauce -- 119
Lea & Perrins -- 115
Mayonnaise (low-fat) -- 93
Mustard (Dijon) -- 160
Mustard (English) -- 167
Mustard (grain) -- 159
Pesto -- 431
Roasted aubergine spread/dip -- 102
Roasted red pepper spread/dip -- 235
Salad dressing (balsamic) -- 209
Salad dressing (Caesar no fat) -- 61
Salad dressing (olive oil and lemon) -- 439
Salad dressing (low-calorie) -- 68
Soy sauce -- 105
Sundried tomatoes -- 167
Taramasalata -- 516
Tartare sauce -- 358
Tikka masala sauce -- 133
Tomato and basil sauce -- 60
Tomato ketchup -- 102
Tzatziki -- 137
Vegemite -- 189
Vinegar (balsamic) -- 138
Vinegar (red wine) -- 23
Vinegar (white wine) -- 22

SWEET
Caramel sauce -- 389
Chocolate sauce -- 367
Cranberry sauce -- 192
Honey -- 334
Icing -- 405
Jam (strawberry) -- 258
Maple syrup -- 265
Marmalade -- 266
Nutella -- 529
Treacle 100G 294 -- 294

SAVOURY SNACKS
Breadsticks -- 408
Cheese straws -- 520
French fries (oven-baked) -- 260
Muffins (blueberry) -- 387
Pizza (Margherita) -- 258
Popcorn (salty) -- 520
Popcorn (sweet) -- 493
Potato chips (ready salted) -- 529
Quiche -- 261
Peanuts (unsalted) -- 561
Salted peanuts -- 621
Salted mixed nuts -- 667
Samosas (vegetable) -- 225
Vege Sausage roll -- 340
Vegetable chips -- 502

SEEDS
Chia seeds -- 422
Hemp seeds -- 437
Pumpkin seeds -- 590
Sesame seeds -- 616
Sunflower seeds -- 591
Flaxseed -- 495

SOUPS – per 100ml liquid
Bouillon -- 7
Carrot and coriander -- 35
 noodle -- 35
Chowder -- 53
Cream of mushroom (Heinz) -- 50
Leek and potato -- 53
Light broth -- 36
Lobster bisque -- 68
Miso -- 22
Onion -- 45
Passata -- 31
Tomato (Heinz) -- 59
Tomato and basil -- 40
Vegetable -- 45

SWEETS
Cadbury's dairy milk -- 525
Green and Black's 70% chocolate -- 575
Green and Black's 85% chocolate -- 630
Haribo -- 344

Hob Nobs – Mcvities -- 473
Jaffa cakes -- 377
Lindt 70% chocolate -- 540
Tic Tacs -- 391
Wine gums -- 325

VEGETABLES
Artichoke (globe) -- 24
Artichoke (Jerusalem) -- 73
Asparagus -- 27
Aubergine
sliced and griddled/grilled -- 18
Avocado -- 193

Beans - green
Trimmed raw -- 24
Trimmed, boiled -- 22
Canned -- 24
Frozen, whole -- 25
Frozen, sliced -- 27
Runner beans, trimmed, boiled -- 18

Bean sprouts -- 32
Beetroot -- 38

Bok Choy -- 15

Broad beans
Canned -- 82

Frozen, boiled -- 81
Fresh, shelled -- 77

Broccoli -- 32
Brussel sprouts -- 43
Cabbage -- 29
Carrot -- 34
Cauliflower -- 35
Celeriac -- 17
Celery -- 8
Chard -- 17
Chicory -- 19
Corn - see Sweetcorn
Courgette -- 18
Cucumber -- 10
Endive -- 17
Fennel -- 14
Garlic -- 106
Kale -- 33
Leeks -- 23

Lettuce -- 15
Hearts of Romaine -- 16
Iceberg -- 14
Mediterranean mixed -- 19
Mixed leaf -- 17
Rocket -- 24
Round -- 15

Mushrooms
Closed cup -- 16
Oyster -- 8
Portobello -- 13
Shiitake -- 27
Shiitake Dried -- 296

Onion (red) -- 38
Onion (white) -- 38
Peas, garden (frozen) -- 86
Peas, petit pois -- 52

Peppers
Chilli, green -- 20
Green, stalk & seeds removed -- 15
Jalapenos, green, sliced -- 24
Jalapenos, red, sliced -- 69
Mixed peppers, sliced, frozen -- 28
Red, stalk & seeds removed -- 32
Yellow, stalk & seeds removed -- 26

Potato (white) -- 79
Radicchio -- 19
Radish -- 13
Radish White (Mooli) -- 15
Ratatouille canned -- 50
Spinach -- 25
Spinach frozen, boiled -- 21
Squash -- 40

Sweetcorn
Giant baby cobs green giant -- 28
Mini corncobs canned -- 23
Mini corncobs fresh/frozen boiled -- 24
On the cob -- 110

Sweetcorn kernels
Canned, drained, re-heated -- 122
Frozen -- 93
Nib lets with peppers (Green Giant) -- 82
Nib lets, canned (Green Giant) -- 100
Nib lets, natur sweet (Green Giant) -- 77
Nib lets, salad crisp (Green Giant) -- 70

Sweet potatoes -- 93
Swiss chard -- 19
Tomato -- 20
Turnip -- 24
Watercress -- 26

Meat Substitute
Tofu -- 70
Quorn (chunky-style pieces) -- 114
Cauldron sausages -- 163
Veggie burgers -- 137

ABOUT THE AUTHOR

Liz Armond is a bestselling author, born and educated in London, UK. She has been an active student of fitness and nutrition for over 30 years. She has always tried to lead a healthy lifestyle and is constantly looking for ways to get healthier and live longer.

After trying out the 5.2 diet with great success she put together her favorite recipes adapted for the 5:2 and published her complete series of cookbooks suitable for every diet.

Liz is now an enthusiastic advocate for this proven diet and is a firm believer that following this diet and maintaining a healthy lifestyle will achieve her goal of living a long and happy life.

She is married with two children and is an enthusiastic golfer, rambler and is keen but not yet proficient in yoga and meditation. She also loves to ski whenever possible.

OTHER BOOKS BY LIZ ARMOND

5:2 Fast Diet Series
Recipes for the 5:2 Fast Diet
The Fast Diet Cookbook
Vegetarian Recipes for the 5:2 Fast Diet
Gluten Free Recipes for the 5:2 Fast Diet
Vegetarian and Gluten Free for the 5:2 Fast Diet
Breakfast Recipes for the 5:2 Fast Diet
Meal Plans & Recipes for the 5:2 Diet
Vegetarian Meal Plans for the 5:2 Diet
Meals for One for the 5:2 Fast Diet
Vegetarian Single Meals for the 5:2 Fast Diet

Other
Fasting Your Way to Health

ONE FINAL THING

If you believe the book is worth sharing, I would be eternally grateful if you could take a few seconds to leave an honest review or to let your friends know about it through Facebook and Twitter.

If it turns out to make a difference in their lives, they will be forever grateful to you, as will I.

All the very best and good luck with all the aims in your life and your successful weight loss.

Liz Armond

Website: - http://lizarmond.com